CONQUERING GERD

A COMPREHENSIVE GUIDE TO UNDERSTANDING GASTROESOPHAGEAL REFLUX DISEASE

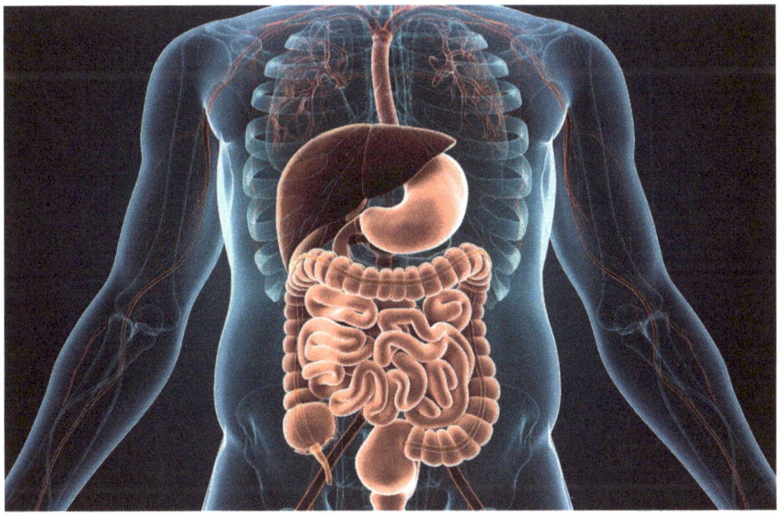

Take Control Of Your Digestive Health

By Delatria Sam

Conquering GERD: A Comprehensive Guide To Understanding Gastroesophageal Reflux Disease

ISBN: 979-8-2954-1178-6

DEDICATED TO

the brave individuals living with GERD,
their caregivers, and loved ones,
who face each day with courage and resilience.

May this book be hope,
a source of comfort, and a guide on your journey
towards healing, wellness, and a life free from the burdens of GERD.

To those who have struggled, and those who continue to strive,
may these pages offer solace, understanding, and practical
wisdom.

To the caregivers, who walk alongside,
may this book provide support, encouragement, and a reminder
that you are not alone in this journey.

With love, empathy, and a deep understanding,
this book is dedicated to you,
and to the countless individuals who have shared their stories,
hopes, and dreams with me.

May we all find peace, healing, and a brighter future,
free from the grip of GERD.

With love and support,

Delatria Sam

WHAT IS GERD?

GERD stands for Gastroesophageal Reflux Disease. It's a chronic condition where stomach acid flows back into the esophagus, causing symptoms like heartburn, chest pain, and difficulty swallowing.

MOST COMMON SYMPTOMS:

- Heartburn (chest pain or discomfort)
- Regurgitation (food or acid returning to the mouth)
- Difficulty swallowing (dysphagia)
- Chest pain or pressure
- Bloating and gas
- Nausea and vomiting
- Coughing or wheezing
- Hoarseness or a sour taste in the mouth

WHO'S AT RISK:

- People over 40
- Those who are overweight or obese
- Pregnant women
- Smokers
- People who eat large meals or lie down after eating
- Those who consume trigger foods like citrus, tomatoes, chocolate, or spicy foods
- People with a hiatal hernia
- Those taking certain medications, like antihistamines or painkillers
- Babies born prematurely can be at risk for GERD due to an immature digestive system

WHAT TO DO:

- Talk to a healthcare professional for a proper diagnosis and treatment
- Make lifestyle changes:
- Eat smaller, more frequent meals
- Avoid trigger foods and drinks
- Lose weight if needed
- Elevate the head of your bed
- Avoid lying down after meals
- Consider over-the-counter medications like antacids or acid reducers
- If symptoms persist, your doctor may prescribe stronger medications or recommend further testing

Read Patient's Journey & Caregiver Stories

A Mom's Journey

“My daughter was born premature and struggled with GERD. We thought it was just colic, but it turned out to be reflux. Physical therapy and smaller feedings helped her thrive.”

A Wake-Up Call

"After years of heartburn, I was diagnosed with GERD. Cutting out trigger foods and taking meds has made a huge difference. I wish I'd taken it seriously sooner."

Supporting My Partner

"My partner's GERD flares up when stressed. I've learned to make GERD-friendly meals and encourage relaxation techniques. It's a team effort."

NICU Experience

"Working in the NICU, I saw many premature babies with GERD. It's amazing how tiny patients can thrive with proper care and feeding strategies."

Finding Relief

"I was skeptical about lifestyle changes, but elevating my bed and avoiding triggers really helped my GERD symptoms."

The Emotional Toll

"GERD can be isolating. I felt embarrassed about my symptoms, but talking to others and joining a support group helped me cope."

A Family Affair

"My whole family has GERD. We've learned to cook GERD-friendly meals and support each other through flare-ups."

From Diagnosis to Management

"After a GERD diagnosis, I changed my diet and exercise routine. It's been a journey, but I'm managing my symptoms."

The Importance of Advocacy

"My uncle's GERD went untreated, and he developed complications. Now, I advocate for regular check-ups and screenings."

Finding What Works

"I've tried various treatments for GERD. What works is different for everyone – it's about finding the right combination for you."

Q&A Time

QUESTION

Are there any specific foods that trigger GERD symptoms?

ANSWER

Common trigger foods include citrus fruits, tomatoes, chocolate, spicy foods, and foods high in fat or fried. Keep a food diary to identify your triggers.

5 Foods To Consider To Help Alleviate Symptoms

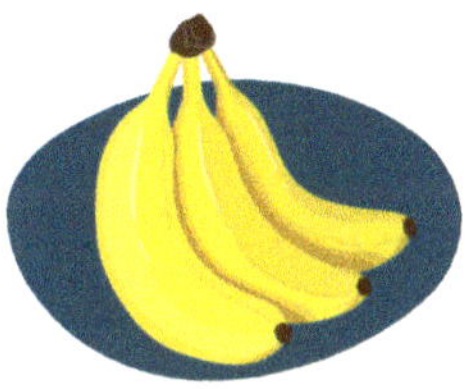

Non-Citrus Fruits

Can reduce irritation and symptoms

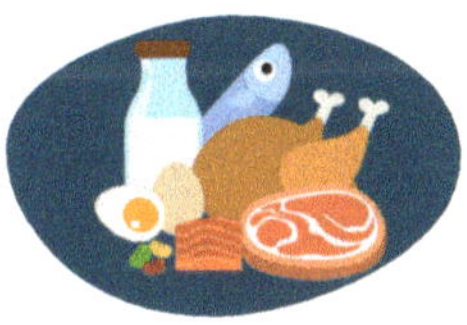

Lean Protein

chicken or fish: Easier to digest, reducing strain on the digestive system and potentially lowering symptom triggers.

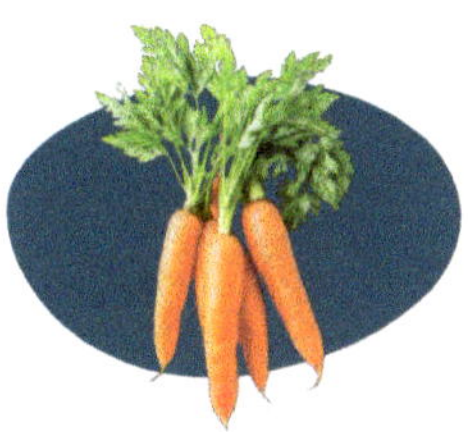

Green beans or carrots

Generally low in fat and less likely to trigger symptoms.

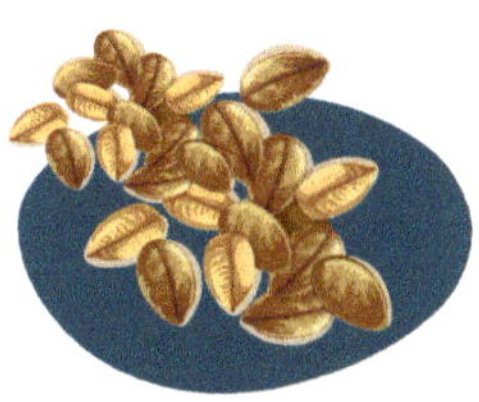

Whole grains like oatmeal

Can aid digestion and are often gentle on the stomach.

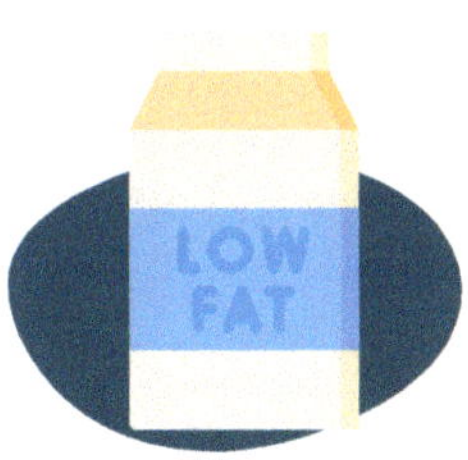

Low-Fat

Lower fat content can reduce relaxation of the lower esophageal sphincter, minimizing reflux.

FOOD DIARY

MONTH: YEAR:

DATE	FOOD/ DRINK	PORTION SIZE	TIME EATEN	SYMPTOMS	TIME

How Is GERD...

Diagnosed?

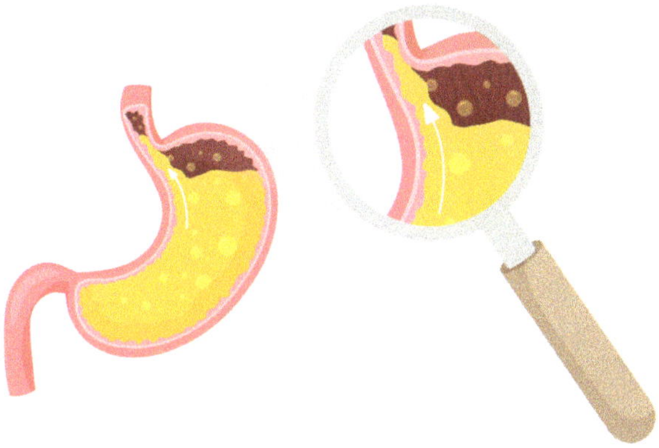

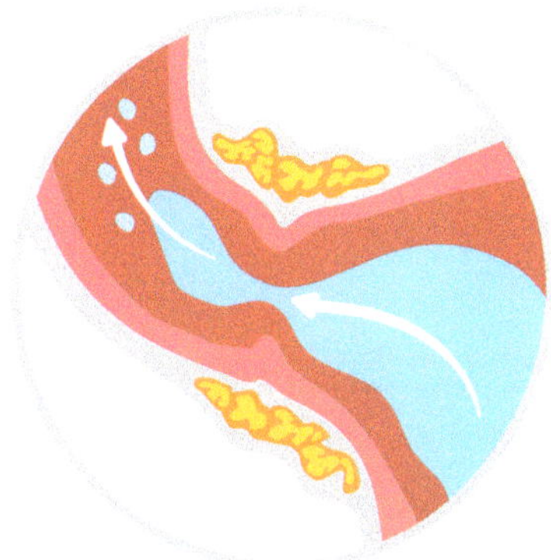

GERD diagnosis typically involves a combination of the following. These tests help rule out other conditions and confirm GERD diagnosis. Your doctor may also recommend lifestyle changes or medication before testing.

✦ Diagnosis

- **Medical History:** Your doctor will ask about symptoms, medical history, and lifestyle habits.
- **Physical Exam:** A physical exam to check for signs of GERD, such as a hiatal hernia.
- **Upper Endoscopy:** A flexible tube with a camera is inserted through the mouth to visualize the esophagus and stomach.
- **Ambulatory Acid Probe Tests:** A probe measures acid levels in the esophagus over 24 hours.
- **Esophageal pH Monitoring:** Measures acid levels in the esophagus over a longer period.
- **Barium Swallow:** A special liquid is swallowed, and X-rays are taken to visualize the esophagus and stomach.
- **Esophageal Manometry:** Measures muscle contractions in the esophagus.

Q&A Time

QUESTION

What can a caregiver or loved one do if they suspect their elderly parent may have symptoms of GERD?

ANSWER

Monitor their symptoms, consult their healthcare provider, and offer support with lifestyle changes like dietary modifications and medication management.

Medication Management Tracker

Date	Medication	Dose	Frequency	Time

Q&A Time

QUESTION

What can a first-time parent do if they suspect their baby may have symptoms of GERD?

ANSWER

Keep a symptom journal, consult your pediatrician, and try soothing techniques like burping, upright positioning, and smaller feedings.

Baby Symptom Journal

Date	Feed	Symptom	Position	Time

Q&A Time

QUESTION

Can GERD lead to complications if left untreated?

ANSWER

Yes, untreated GERD can lead to complications like esophagitis, Barrett's esophagus, and an increased risk of esophageal cancer.

Do's & Don'ts

- **Eat smaller meals:** To reduce pressure on the stomach.
- **Avoid lying down after meals:** Wait a few hours before lying down.
- **Elevate the head of your bed:** To reduce nighttime symptoms.
- **Avoid trigger foods:** Like citrus fruits, tomatoes, chocolate, or spicy foods.

- **Don't** eat large meals before bedtime
- **Don't** consume foods that trigger symptoms
- **Don't** lie down after eating
- **Don't** wear tight clothing that puts pressure on the stomach
- **Don't** ignore symptoms or let them get worse.

MANAGING GERD: 4 HELPFUL TIPS

01 Consider probiotics to help with digestion and symptom management.

02 Chew your food well. It helps with digestion and reduces symptoms.

03 Manage stress: Stress can trigger or worsen GERD symptoms.

04 Avoid caffeine and chocolate.

05 Try Ginger: Ginger has natural anti-inflammatory properties.

Q&A Time

QUESTION

What are some other common symptoms of GERD?

ANSWER

Some other common symptoms of GERD are sleep disturbances, Laryngitis or sore throat, and chronic cough.

DID YOU KNOW?

GERD can affect voice and speech: Acid reflux can cause hoarseness or voice changes.

DID YOU KNOW?

GERD is a global health issue: GERD affects millions of people worldwide, with varying prevalence rates in different populations.

4 Ways To Support Someone Who Has GERD

Encourage dietary changes

Support them in making dietary adjustments like avoiding trigger foods

Help manage stress

Stress can exacerbate GERD symptoms; encourage stress-reducing activities like meditation or yoga.

Support lifestyle adjustments

Encourage habits like eating smaller meals, not lying down after meals, and elevating the head of the bed.

Encourage medical follow-up

Support them in managing their condition with their healthcare provider and following treatment plans.

THOUGHTFUL *gift Ideas*

- ○ Gourmet food basket
- ○ A thoughtful notebook for writing or reflection
- ○ Book by their favorite author
- ○ Relaxation spa kit
- ○ Fitness tracker or smartwatch
- ○ Art piece
- ○ Cozy throw blanket
- ○ Personalized mug
- ○ Handmade craft
- ○ Essential oils or scented candles
- ○ Tech gadget

- ○ Wellness kit
- ○ Personalized planner
- ○ Indoor plant
- ○ Heartfelt letter
- ○ Cookbook
- ○ Hot & cold therapy packs
- ○ Heating pads
- ○ Crossword puzzles
- ○ Tablet or e-reader
- ○ Coloring books
- ○ Flowers
- ○ Humiidifer
- ○ Sound machine
- ○ Health magazine
- ○ Bottled water
- ○ Organizer

CONVERSATION BETWEEN A PATIENT AND A DOCTOR REGARDING THE PATIENT'S CONCERN ABOUT GERD:

PATIENT: "I've been having some issues with heartburn and acid reflux lately. I'm worried it might be GERD. Can you help me understand what's going on?"

DOCTOR: "Sure. So, you've been experiencing heartburn and acid reflux symptoms. How often are you experiencing these symptoms, and do you notice any triggers?"

PATIENT: "It's been happening a couple of times a week, usually after I eat big meals or spicy food. Sometimes it wakes me up at night. I've also been having a bit of trouble swallowing sometimes."

DOCTOR: "Okay. Based on what you're describing, it sounds like GERD could be a possibility. We'll review your history and maybe run some tests. Have you tried anything to ease the symptoms?"

PATIENT: "I've been trying to avoid spicy food and eat smaller meals. But it's not totally going away."

DOCTOR: "That's a great start. We can talk about lifestyle changes, possible meds, and review your history. An upper endoscopy can help to check your esophagus. Let me know if you have any questions."

PATIENT: "Sounds good. What can I expect in terms of treatment if it is GERD?"

DOCTOR: "If it's GERD, we'll start meds to reduce acid and discuss diet and lifestyle changes to ease symptoms."

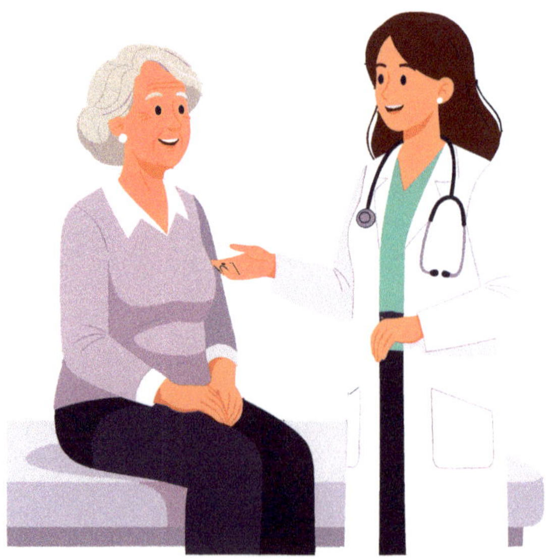

How can I support someone whose living with GERD?

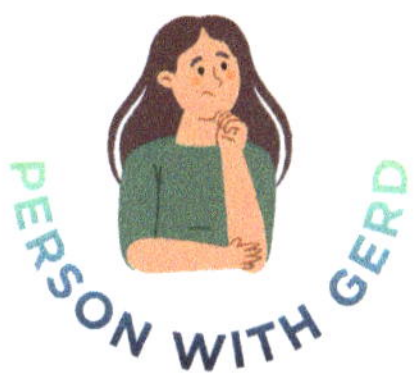

"Hey, I've been dealing with some bad GERD symptoms lately. It's messing with my food choices and sleep."

"Sorry to hear this! What can I do to help? Do you need help cookin' up some GERD-friendly meals or anything?"

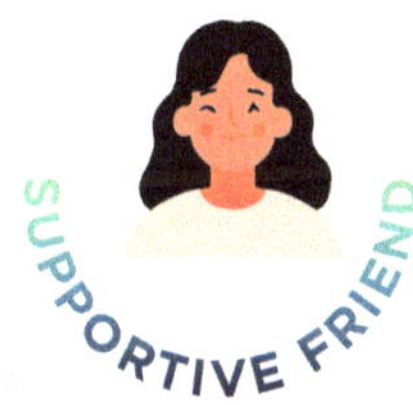

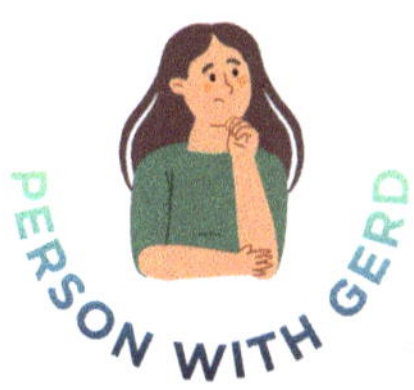

"Yes, that'd be awesome! Avoidin' spicy food and big meals before bed helps a lot. And maybe just checkin' in on me when I'm havin' a rough day?"

"For sure! I'll make sure to prepare some gentle foods for you. And I'll definitely check in on you when you're feeling off. Want me to help you find some good resources on managing GERD, too?"

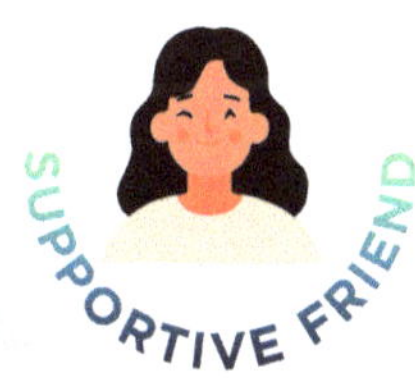

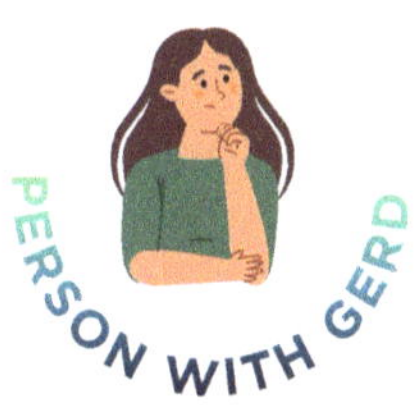

"That'd be super helpful, thanks for being so supportive."

"Of course!"

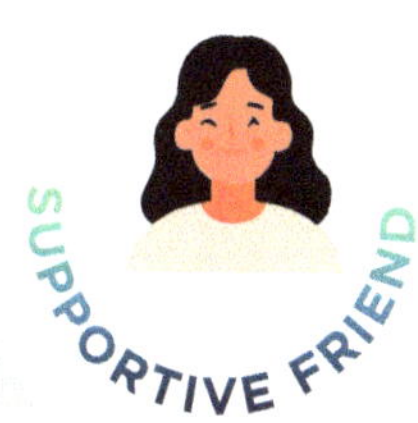

Let's Talk:
GERD
Conversation Starters

How to support someone in the workplace who's living with GERD.

Ask how they're really doing to understand their experience with GERD.

Check if there's anything you can do to support them, like adjusting work schedules or providing stress management resources.

Show interest in what's been on their mind lately to help them feel heard.

Invite them to chat about their needs or concerns regarding GERD in the workplace.

Is there anything we can do to support you?

Start the conversation. Support each other.
Together, we build a healthier workplace.

I listen to my body!

am in control of my health!

I prioritize my well-being!

I adapt and thrive!

I am gentle with myself!

I manage my GERD with care!

Research UPDATE

Lifestyle Modifications

Studies suggest that dietary changes, such as low-carbohydrate diets, can reduce esophageal acid exposure and alleviate symptoms.

GERD has been linked to various conditions, including asthma exacerbations, anxiety, and depression.

Love Letters

Dear Supportive friend

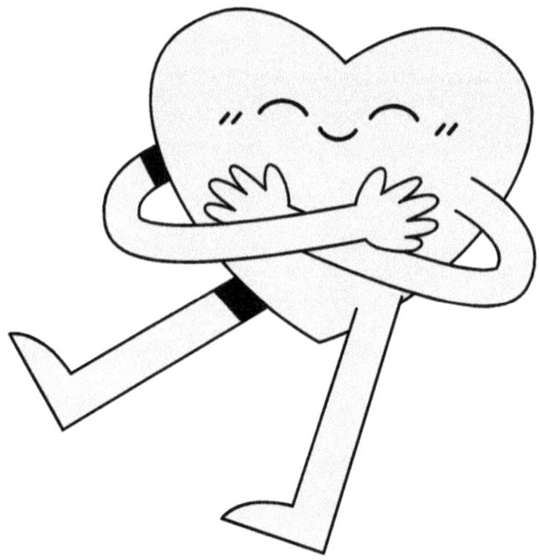

Thank you for listening and being there during tough times. Your care means everything. Thank you for putting up with me. Excuse me if I was ever rude to you. Excuse my lack of knowledge, excuse if sometimes I wanted to give up and didn't want your help. Excuse me for yelling at you and not showing my appreciation.

I love you with all
my heart,

xoxo

To my loving family

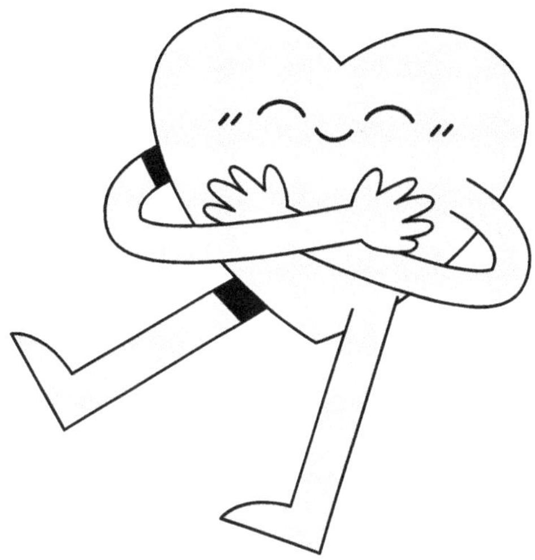

Thanks for understanding and supporting me through GERD challenges. I love you.

I love you with all my heart,

xoxo

Dear
Nurse/Healthcare
Team

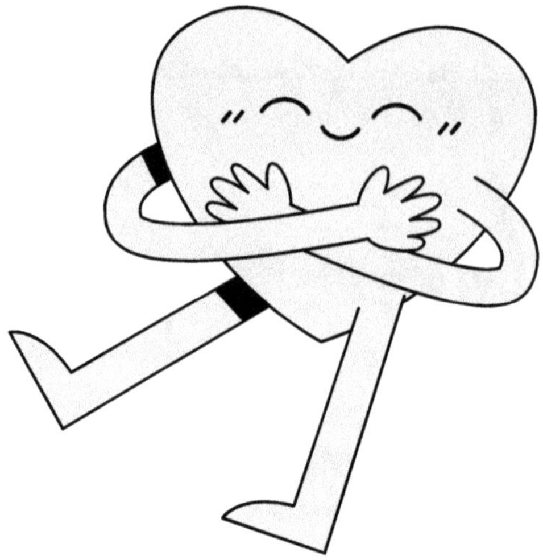

Your expertise and kindness helped me manage GERD.

I love you with all
my heart,

xoxo

Dear Pastor/Church Community

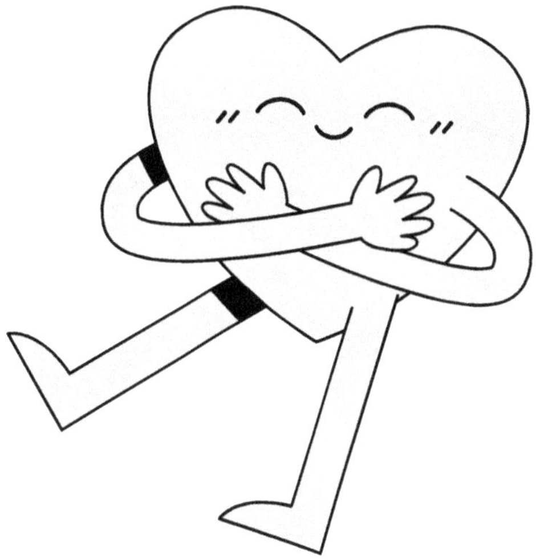

Your prayers and support lifted me. Thank you for being a blessing.

I love you with all my heart,

xoxo

To a Supportive Neighbor

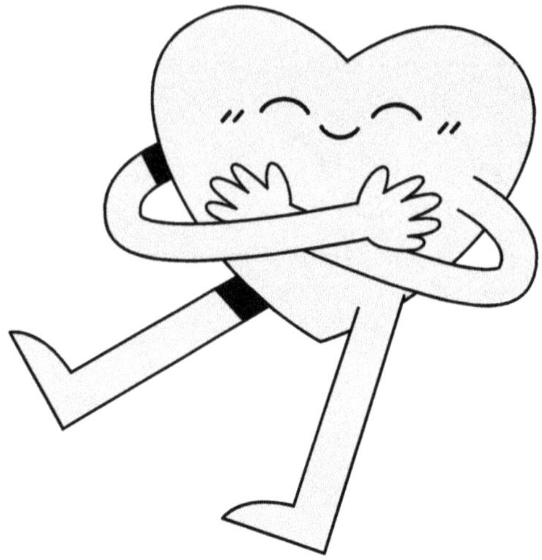

Thanks for checking in and helping when I needed it. You made a difference.

*I love you with all
my heart,*

xoxo

Dear Companion

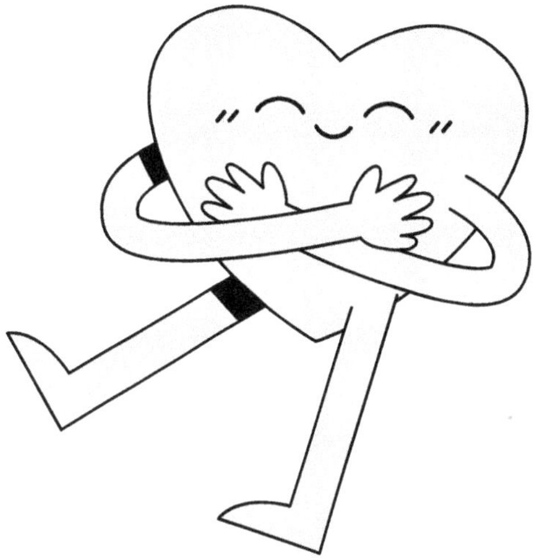

Thanks for standing by me and encouraging me to take care of myself.

I love you with all
my heart,

xoxo

To a Helpful Colleague

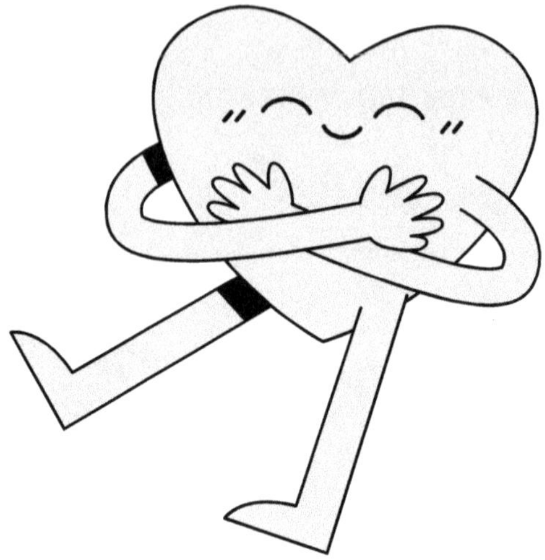

Thanks for adjusting work tasks and being understanding about GERD needs.

I love you with all my heart,

xoxo

Dear Mentor/Writing Coach

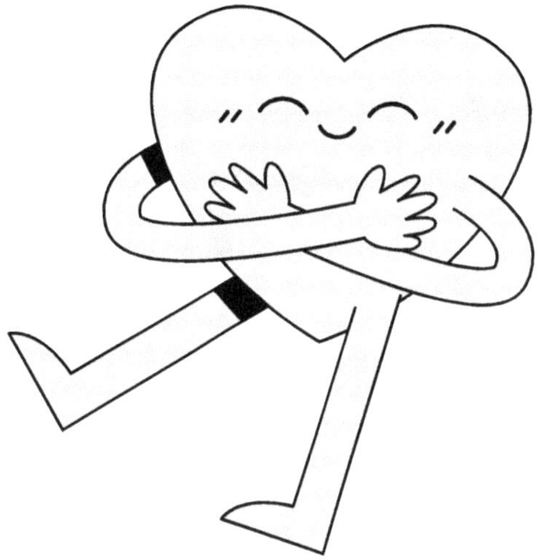

Thanks for encouraging me to share my story and supporting my health journey.

I love you with all
my heart,

xoxo

To my Grandma

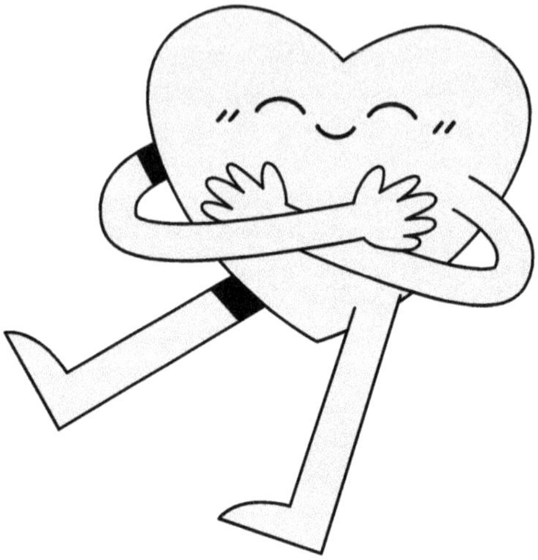

Thanks for your love and prayers. You inspire me to stay positive.

I love you with all my heart,

xoxo

To Everyone who Supported Me

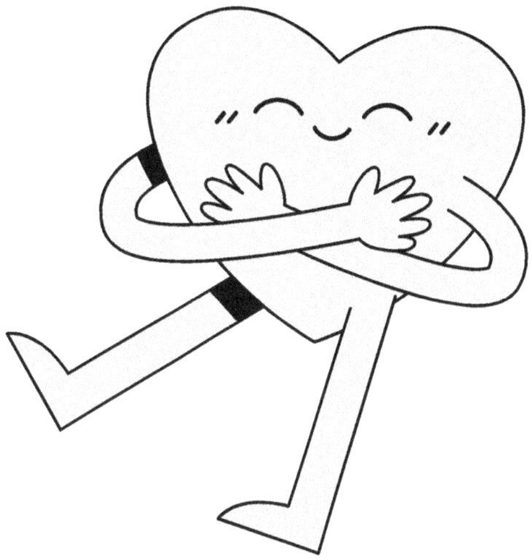

Thanks for being part of my journey. Your kindness and support mean the world.

I love you with all
my heart,

xoxo

www.ingramcontent.com/pod-product-compliance
Lightning Source LLC
LaVergne TN
LVHW070858210926
848482LV00016B/971